CALMING YOUR FUSSY BABY
The
Brazelton Way

also by T. Berry Brazelton, M.D.

On Becoming a Family
The Growth of Attachment Before and After Birth

Infants and Mothers
Differences in Development

Toddlers and Parents
Declaration of Independence

Doctor and Child

To Listen to a Child
Understanding the Normal Problems of Growing Up

Working and Caring

What Every Baby Knows

Families, Crisis, and Caring

Touchpoints
Your Child's Emotional and Behavioral Development

Going to the Doctor

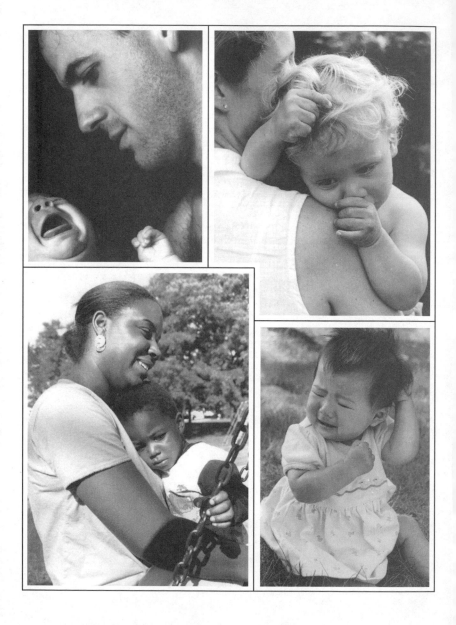

CALMING YOUR FUSSY BABY
The
Brazelton Way

T. Berry Brazelton, M.D.
Joshua D. Sparrow, M.D.

A Merloyd Lawrence Book
PERSEUS PUBLISHING
A Member of the Perseus Books Group

PHOTO CREDITS

**Photographs on title page [upper right and lower right]
by Janice Fullman**

**Photographs on pages xiv, 12 and title page [upper left]
by Dorothy Littell Greco**

**Photographs on page 68 and title page [lower left]
by Marilyn Nolt**

Library of Congress Control Number: 2002114511
ISBN 0–7382–0781–0

Perseus Publishing is a Member of the Perseus Books Group.
Find us on the World Wide Web at http://www.perseuspublishing.com.

Perseus Publishing books are available at special discounts for bulk purchases in the U.S. by corporations, institutions, and other organizations. For more information, please contact the Special Markets Department at the Perseus Books Group, 11 Cambridge Center, Cambridge, MA 02142, or call (800) 255-1514 or (617) 252-5298, or e-mail j.mccrary@perseusbooks.com.

Text design by Trish Wilkinson
Set in 11-point AGaramond by the Perseus Books Group

First printing, January 2003
1 2 3 4 5 6 7 8 9 10—06 05 04 03

To the children and parents
who have taught us so much through the years

Contents

Preface

Ever since the first *Touchpoints* book was published in 1992, I have been asked by parents and professionals all over the country to write some short, practical books about the common challenges that parents face as they raise their children. Among the most common are crying, discipline, and getting a baby or child to sleep, topics that we address in this Brazelton Way series.

In my years of pediatric practice, families have taught me that problems in these areas often arise predictably as a child develops. In these short books I have tried to address the problems with crying, discipline, and sleep that parents are bound to encounter as their children regress just before they make their next developmental leap. Each book describes these "touchpoints" of crying, discipline, or sleep, so that parents can better understand their child's behavior. Each also offers practical suggestions on how parents can help children master the particular challenges they face in these areas and get back on track.

As with *Touchpoints Three to Six*, I have invited Joshua Sparrow, M.D., to co-author these books with me, to add his perspective as a child psychiatrist. In general, these books focus on the concerns and opportunities of the first six years of life, though occasionally we refer to older children's issues. In a final chapter of each book, special problems are discussed, though these short books are not intended to cover these topics exhaustively, nor are they meant to replace firsthand professional diagnosis and treatment. Instead, we hope that these books will serve as easy-to-use guides for parents to turn to as they face their child's growing pains, or the "touchpoints" that signal exciting leaps of development.

Though difficulties such as "colic" or excessive crying, middle of the night wakings, or temper tantrums, for example, are both common and predictable, they make great demands on parents. These kinds of problems are for the most part temporary and not serious. Yet without support and understanding, a family can be overwhelmed, and a child's development can veer seriously off course. It is our hope that the straightforward information provided in these books will help prevent those unnecessary derailments and provide reassurance for parents in times of uncertainty, so that even in those challenging moments, the excitement and joy of helping a young child grow can be rekindled.

CALMING YOUR FUSSY BABY
The
Brazelton Way

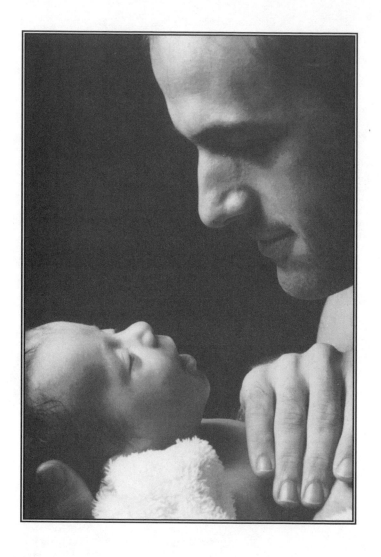

CHAPTER 1

Your Baby's Language

How Your Baby Communicates

The most expectable question I receive as a pediatrician from new parents as they prepare to take their newborn baby home is, "How will I ever know how to nurture this baby? How will I know what she wants and needs?"

My answer is, "Learn to watch your baby. Her behavior will guide you. When she likes what you are doing, she'll tell you with her face and her whole body. She'll brighten, her body will wiggle, and her arms and legs will reach out. When she doesn't, it will be just as apparent. She'll stiffen, turn away, and begin to fuss or to cry. Babies give you clear cues, if you are watching for them."

"But how will I know how to keep from making mistakes?"

"You won't. Learning to parent is learning from mistakes. In fact, you learn more from your mistakes than you do from successes."

Since every parent wants to "do it right," my best advice is to learn the language of your baby. Her behavior is her language.

The test that I designed for new babies (the Neonatal Behavioral Assessment Scale, NBAS; see the www.brazelton-institute.com Web site for information on the new, shorter CLNBAS) allows a newborn baby's behavior to be "read" and shared with parents. By watching—with a trained observer—the baby's responses to sights, sounds, and other sensations, and watching her move from sleeping to an alert state, new parents can discover many aspects of their newborn's personality, or temperament. The baby's amazing skills can be pointed out by a trained nurse, doctor, or other healthcare professional to help alert parents to ways of handling their new baby. With my scale, parents can watch their newborn shut out disturbing sensations, come awake, and respond to a rattle, to a red ball, and to a human face. They can learn what to expect, and what behavior they may be able to shape or not—when to feed and when to let the newborn sleep. Right from the first parents can learn to understand the way different babies respond to the world, whether a quiet, sensitive baby, a very active, driving baby, or any baby in between.

When parents get a chance to watch all of these different kinds of behavior in the newborn nursery, they can begin to understand their baby as a person. These responses in the nursery can be a model for parents when they start out at home with their newborn. Hospital stays for labor and delivery are so short these days that expectant parents might ask ahead for this kind of demonstration. New parents bring so much passion to getting to know their new baby. Soon both they and the baby begin to fall in love. Now they can start to fit their hopes and experience to the individuality of their baby as a person.

Crying

Crying is the most powerful of a newborn's communications. No other signal matches the power of crying in reaching parents.

A newborn baby announces her arrival with a cry. The first cry serves many purposes:

- it opens the lungs and brings them into action,
- it helps empty the fluid in the baby's airways so oxygen can be absorbed, and
- it is an important part of the infant's stress response that gets her survival outside the mother's body started.

With that first cry comes a massive startle. Legs and arms flail. All of this mobilizes everyone present at the delivery to pay attention. The baby's face scrunches up as if to say, "I am here! Take care of me!"

From that moment on, crying has a special meaning for parents and caretakers of that small baby. Can you hear a small baby's cry without feeling your heart speed up, without an urge to pick that baby up and comfort her? It's built into all of us as an "instinctive" response—to protect and nurture the smallest, most vulnerable member of our species.

Meeting the demands of a newborn's cry is one of the first challenges for new parents. Is she hungry? Is she uncomfortable? Does she need to be changed? Is she tired or bored? Or, could she be in real pain? All of these are questions that set off an "alarm reaction" in new parents, forcing them to search for a solution.

Smiling

The fetus has been "smiling" in the uterus, even before birth. Or is it a frown? When we watch 7-month fetuses by ultrasound, we have seen their lips spread as in a smile, but without a change in their face. This happens as the fetus shifts from a deeper sleep into a lighter sleep state. So, it is no surprise that parents report that their newborn babies are seen to smile as they begin to wake up or go to sleep. This "smiling" seems to be a response to the change in sleep-awake states. Parents will be excited by it and are likely to reinforce any smile or frown with an immediate positive response. Of course, this response from parents rewards the behavior for the baby and she is more likely to want to repeat it.

In the first month, the smile may begin to appear in several different situations. As her face and eyes become more mobile, and begin to move in coordination with her mouth, parents are likely to say, "Look at her. She's trying to smile!" They cuddle her. They stroke her. They coo to her to get another. Even before we can expect a "real" smile at 4 to 6 weeks, they are preparing the way. By 6 weeks she smiles in response to her parents' coos and cuddles: This has become an expected way of communicating. When a baby smiles, her parents nearly faint with pleasure. If they react too strongly, she is likely to suppress the smile. If, on the other hand, they can croon softly to her or they can hold her tenderly, to rock her or sing to her, they are reinforcing the positive social aspect of her smile. She will very quickly learn that this is another way to bring important people to her.

Body Language

A baby's body language is another source of information. When you diaper her, and lean over her to talk and to coo, watch as she listens, "cycling" with her legs and arms. She chortles with her voice, but her body tells you as much about her delight. When you pick her up at the wrong time, her whole body stiffens. Her legs and arms become rigid or jerky. Her hands stiffen into fists, and her neck arches as she turns her head and eyes away.

When you cuddle her in your arms, her body softens and curls up around you. She turns her head into your chest, or she looks up intently into your face, her hands clutching at your clothing or your finger. When she is comfortable, her legs droop, but they droop around you. Her body is carefully adjusting to yours. Up on your shoulder, she lifts her head to look around, and her legs even clasp around you. As she looks around the room she finally relaxes to put her soft little head in the corner of your neck. She and you have communicated. She seems to say "this is where I feel safe and cared for." Nursing mothers let milk down at this point—it is such a delicious experience.

Eye Contact

Right from the first, the newborn baby comes from sleep or crying to an alert state. Often a parent or a nurse might tilt the baby up to a 30 degree angle, holding onto her arms and even a leg, to keep her from startling. For when she startles, she becomes upset and can't concentrate. But watch the new baby when she begins to concentrate on looking. She keeps herself under control as she looks. She almost arches forward as she works to stare at your face. If you move slowly, with your face about a foot away and just ahead of hers, she will follow your face. She works hard to concentrate on a person who leans over her. Her bright eyes almost leap out of her head to draw you in. She says, "I'm here! I'm a person! Love me." Her eyes almost speak for her. Eye-to-eye contact can be so exciting!

As she gets older, her control over her body and her ability to focus and follow increase.

She can use this ability to communicate with you. Her eyes say so much. "I want you! I'm tired. Help me." Even "feed me." Though every new parent says, "How will I understand her," your baby's eyes will tell you what she needs. When they are bright and loving, her eyes say, "You are my parent and you are just right!"

"Too Much"

Every baby reaches a point beyond which any new information or experience is too much. When she has had too much, she has many ways to say "that's enough." Arching, turning her eyes and face away, or her face going pale.

With her eyes half shut, she may even hiccup, spit up, or have a noisy bowel movement. All of these can be signals that she has had enough for the moment—enough sights and sounds, enough playing and interaction. She may be tired and need a nap before she'll be ready for more. Many babies will react this way to a noisy or crowded room. This may be why she goes to sleep at grandma's. Too many people, too much attention, and she must "tune out." Take her reactions seriously, and shelter her from too many sensations. After a quiet period of recovery, she may be ready to interact all over again. This is protective behavior. This may be her only way of letting you know she's had enough.

Sucking

A small baby tells you so much by her sucking. When she needs comfort, she turns to her mother's breast to suck (not just for food, but for comfort). When she is resourceful, she can turn to her own fingers to comfort and soothe herself. When she's hungry, she'll suck steadily. But as soon as her initial hunger is satisfied, she will fall into a pattern of a burst of sucking followed by a pause, then more burst-pause-burst. Parents will jiggle the baby to keep eating, or look down at her face to say "Keep going!" But the baby is using these pauses for communication, to look up into your face and to learn about you. The pace of sucking at feeding time seems set up to make time for looking and listening.

There are two kinds of sucking—sucking for food, and another kind for "place-holding." In "place-holding" the sucking is concentrated in the top of the baby's mouth (you can feel it yourself when you let your baby suck on your finger). This "place-holding" sucking is used to pacify, to settle the body's movements, to concentrate on listening or looking, to go to sleep, or even to wake up from sleep more gently. A baby's sucking says a lot, if you watch, and listen.

Self-Soothing

As a new baby lies in her crib, she begins to squirm. Sleeping on her back, she is likely to throw off a startle. The startle will upset her. She may start crying, and may startle again, with her cry increasing in tempo. As she loses control, she will use four reflexes to retain control over herself. She will turn her head to one side, her face and arm stretch out, and her body arches away from her face side. She has produced a tonic neck reflex. This in turn leads to a hand brought up to her mouth (called a Babkin hand-to-mouth reflex). She roots around the hand, head turning from side to side. Finally, she gets a thumb or her fingers into her mouth to suck on them. The fourth reflex is now accomplished and she has gotten herself under control.

Now, she can look and listen and can begin to learn about her new world! She has calmed herself down—a first step in self-control, and a major achievement! Any adoring parent will lean over her to say softly, "That was wonderful!" And it was! The baby knows her new self-control is wonderful too. She sucks her thumb keenly, but may also let out a soft sound of contentment. Her parent coos to her. She tries to coo back, but can't—yet. She extracts her thumb, looks bright-eyed toward her softly vocalizing parent. She wriggles with contentment. But no sound comes.

Cooing

In another few weeks, she can begin to murmur or to coo as she wriggles. This form of communication usually begins to surface when the baby is about three months old. She finds her parents even more responsive as the new sounds she makes become a part of the wriggle. In the next few months, she will practice them as she lies in bed. Over and over she gurgles, coos, even lets out a loud sound. She is learning how to gain control over these thrilling new achievements. Often, she will startle to her own sounds. She is excited and may lose control in crying, which brings her parent to her. As soon as her parent arrives, the crying stops. She looks up to smile, to coo, to wriggle content-edly—hoping to keep her parent there.

"Getting It Right"

There are few instances when a parent of a young child feels "I got it right! I did the right thing!" Maybe a big burp. But satisfying a child's crying by understanding what's going on inside her head and responding appropri-ately is always one of those. "I am her parent—and I know what to do when she needs me." What a triumph! We hope this book will help parents achieve more of those triumphs.

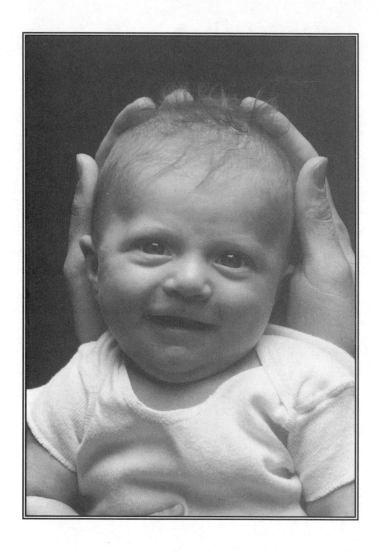

CHAPTER 2

Touchpoints of Communication

Newborn Crying

Recognizing a Newborn's Cries

A new mother may be able to recognize her own baby's cry in a crowded nursery within the first three days! She will have become so attuned, so passionately ready to satisfy her newborn.

The passion that new mothers and fathers bring to a newborn may lead them to recognize and distinguish between different cries of their newborn by three weeks of age. Parents also use their infant's facial expressions, body language, and other information (time of last feeding, nap, or diaper change, noise, bright lights, too much clothing or too little, for example) to understand what each cry is saying. Of course our descriptions of each cry are oversimplified here, but see if you can begin to recognize your baby's different cries.

Pain.   A cry of pain is a short, loudly piercing wail, high-pitched, with a period of apnea (no breath), then another wail. This cry does not stop when a baby in pain is comforted or picked up. When a baby in pain cries for a prolonged period, it may begin to sound weaker and less like pain, but it certainly is time to ask your doctor for help. The face is screwed up, the arms, legs, and body are held tightly up against the body. Parents can try to examine the baby for the painful area by pressing all over the body gently. The stomach, the legs and arms, even the head, face, and ears may be cues. Always gently feel the soft spot (fontanel) on top of a baby's head to see whether it is soft between cries. If it is not, it is an urgent signal for help. You can also bend the baby's neck gently and work with the legs and arms to find the source.

The source of the pain must be found. Look for any reason why the baby is crying. Press around—gently—everywhere. If you can't find the reason, you will need to ask your doctor for help.

Knowing the difference between pain cries and other cries is important right from the first. Sometimes a pain cry demands urgent access to a professional for help. All new parents deserve a medical "home" for their infants—a healthcare provider who knows parent and child well, who is personally available to respond to urgent concerns, and who carefully arranges for another professional to be available whenever he or she is not, including evenings and weekends.

Hunger.   A hungry newborn will cry in short, continuous bursts. This crying is insistent, medium in pitch.

A parent can be sure that her baby is hungry when he bobs his head forward and side-to-side, mouth open, on the lookout for bottle or breast. An active baby may even seem to be taking swipes at the air with his searching little lips. Watch as he attempts to bring his hand and bedclothes up to his mouth, as he roots to find a nipple that will feed him!

Whenever a baby cries, a parent's instinct will be to try a feeding first. It rarely goes wrong, and one can see by the baby's rooting behavior how critical sucking and taking in food may be in settling this cry. As the baby sucks, one can see how hungry he was and his satisfaction as he tries to satisfy himself. When another kind of cry is mistaken for hunger, the baby may take the nipple (as if politely), but resort soon again to fussing and looking around.

When the baby is sucking for food, a parent might notice that he starts with a series of forceful sucks. But soon, these will develop into a burst–pause pattern: suck–suck–suck–suck–pause–suck–suck–suck–pause. It is already clear that he is satisfied. He wants to stop to look around and listen, and sets up a rhythm of sucking and stopping. The pauses are interesting times for looking into the faces of those who feed him. Look down at him to smile, to coo and hug him before you push him to go on sucking. The satisfaction and rhythmic pattern brought by sucking helps the baby tune in to his parents.

Fatigue.   When the day has been overloaded with too much handling, too much interaction with others, too much noise or activity around him, a new baby is likely to start protesting. A soft crying, almost a whimper, builds up to a peak of loud distressed cries. When he is put to bed or given a chance to be less stimulated, cries change to sobs, and finally stop. Parents will blame themselves: "Why didn't I put him to sleep before this?" But the baby's ability to protest and settle down is something to be admired.

Boredom.   A bored baby will whimper, in bursts. Searching with his eyes and head, he will stop fussing when he's spoken to, or jostled, or picked up to be played with. Almost anything satisfies him as long as it's something new.

The baby's face is softer, the eyes are usually open though dull. He looks around vaguely, as if searching for something to look at. He stops to listen if there is an interesting sound. His body is more relaxed and his hands are open. Often, his feet wave in the air, as if for exercise. He may even catch sight of one of them and stop his fussing to watch it. His hand comes up to his mouth, but it is not useful, if sucking is not his goal.

Soothing a bored baby is very easy. But it can take time, energy, and patience—all of which can be in short supply for any parent. Pick him up to cuddle and talk to him. He seems satisfied to gaze at a face or a bright toy. Talking to him in a quiet, insistent voice calms him. This is certainly a time to interact and play with him. Carry him around the house or outside. Baby packs or pouches are like the lovely wraps and serapes that many cultures use to keep the baby close and enable enjoyable interactions between parent and child.

Discomfort.   This is a less piercing cry than pain, with forceful bursts of loud crying. The baby seems to be insisting that he is distressed by something, sometimes, a bubble of gas. Intermittent cries that are not too disturbing make this crying easy to distinguish from real pain. For example, when the baby is picked up to see whether the discomfort can be relieved, this low-keyed whimpering usually stops.

Try all the maneuvers suggested above to see whether you can calm the fussing. Press around his body (see *Pain,* above) to try to find a more serious reason. Notice his face: frowning forehead, questioning eyes, legs and arms are tenser than with boredom, but can relax when you examine him.

If no reason is found, offer the baby a feeding, or water, then burp him, and help him suck—on a nipple, or on fingers (yours or his own). Often a bowel movement is on its way. If the discomfort is serious, it will build up to a cry of pain or a more desperate plea for help.

Letting off steam at the end of the day.   This is often mistaken for "colic" or discomfort. The intermittent, often rhythmic fussing cry is usually set off after a busy day of being overloaded with sights, sounds, activity. The rhythm of a low-keyed buildup—fussing, stopping, fussing, stopping—can be temporarily handled by talking to the baby, or picking him up, or rocking him. Although it can build up to a real peak of fussy crying (resembling pain), for the most part it is fussy and rhythmic. The baby's face is soft, frowning a bit, but alternates with relaxation of face and body. Almost any maneuver stops this temporarily but it may resume when you stop. (See also "*Colic*" later in this chapter.)

These different cries may be recognized and parents who are learning about their babies may feel that they can distinguish them as early as three weeks. When a new parent

What To Do When a Baby Cries

1. Try to identify the kind of cry and what the baby's other behaviors are telling you. Use other clues—for example, time of last feeding, last nap, last diaper change, baby's reactions to sounds, light, air temperature, activity, and movement.
2. Change him. Try feeding him. If it is soon after a nursing or a bottle, he probably won't need to be fed again. Still, sucking is a powerful soother. Help him find his fist or thumb. Or let him suck on your finger or sugar water.
3. Speak softly and comfortingly until you break through the crying, then try to bring the pitch and volume of his crying down by slowly lowering your own voice.
4. Hold his arms and body to avoid startles.
5. Swaddle him with his baby blanket, so that his legs and arms are firmly contained. Be sure to place him on his back, and near you, so that you can be sure that he does not snuggle down inside the blanket, where he could possibly suffocate.
6. Pick him up to cuddle.
7. Try massaging his back and limbs gently.
8. Sing to him.
9. Walk with him. Even rock him up and down, or gently swing him.

(continued on next page)

What To Do When a Baby Cries

(continued from previous page)

10. Use white noise or motion. Parents tell me they set their infant on a washing machine, or use a "white noise" machine to soothe him. Some take the baby for a ride in the car. While this may work, crying is likely to start again when the repetitive stimulation stops. It creates a kind of shutting out in small babies that we call "habituation": An infant quiets, even puts himself to sleep, but only to avoid all the commotion. It is likely to work only as long as the repetitious stimulation persists. When the crying starts again, it is usually due to whatever set it off in the first place.

11. Another way to quiet a fussy, unsettled baby is what I call a "football hold." Placing the baby across your forearm on his belly, chest in your hand, legs and arms dangling, your other hand securely on his back, you can gently rock the baby up and down. When he begins to quiet, he'll lift his head and look around. Sing to him and croon comfortingly. As he slows to quiet, use his interest in the world to maintain his quiet alertness. Watch his eyes open wide. Many babies quiet, often because it is more difficult when they are on their bellies to take the deep breaths that are necessary to crying. But the rhythmic rocking and the interesting sights and sounds also help him to maintain his control. This method can offer a short break for desperate parents.

can tell these cries apart, she will begin to know just what her baby needs. What powerful proof of the passion that a new parent brings to this relationship!

All of these maneuvers can be used to reassure oneself that the baby is not in pain, even if nothing seems to stop the crying for long. When the infant does respond to your maneuvers, even temporarily, it can be reassuring.

It is so difficult to have a "hard to read" baby. The signals you ordinarily rely upon aren't there. Learning about that baby is more difficult. Hard to read or not, can you spoil a small baby? Not likely. This kind of attention is the way you are learning how to satisfy your baby.

Each time parents find that their efforts to calm a baby work, they are encouraged by a successful experience. When these don't work, they are likely to try one maneuver after another, often with increasing anxiety and tension. But we all learn most from failures. If you cannot find an immediate solution, it may be time to stop, pull back, and wonder what next—and, in the process, to observe the infant. As you do, you learn more and more about him.

Although I always try to reassure parents of a crying baby that no one takes their baby's cries as seriously as they do, we all tend to respond—and to criticize—parents when their efforts don't work. We are often too ready to "blame the victim" (the mother or father) when a baby cries.

"What are they doing to him? Why don't they help him?" Pressure from other adults adds quickly to a frantic parent's anxiety. Learning how to satisfy a newborn baby's cries can feel like an all-too-urgent challenge to a new parent.

Crying and Temperament

The quality of a newborn's cry and his ability to be soothed give parents two important windows into the baby's future—a window into his temperamental style and into the "work" a parent must do to comfort him. An intense, driving baby is likely to demonstrate a high activity level, a swift buildup to crying, and a loud, high-pitched kind of crying that may be difficult to soothe. A quiet and sensitive baby is likely to be slower to warm up and to have a lower-pitched but insistent wail. He may make repeated attempts to calm himself—by sucking his thumb, looking around, or changing positions. When he finally can't be comforted, his wailing can be insistent and disturbing. These patterns are part of each baby's temperament and style. (I describe these individual differences at some length in *Infants and Mothers*.) They also shape the parents' image of the child and influence the adjustment parents must make as they try to get to know him.

The kind and amount of crying are affected by the baby's temperament, as is his ability to comfort and settle himself. A quiet, watchful baby is likely to combine his cries with attempts to use his eyes, his ears, or even his quiet movements such as his hand-to-mouth and finger sucking. A highly sensitive baby, who startles with each loud sound or sudden change in handling, is likely to use crying as a way of letting off steam, of discharging his easily overloaded nervous system. An active, driving baby will combine his activity and his startles with cycles of loud crying before he stops to return to his active movements. It is as if the crying were all a part of a language with which each different kind of newborn were equipped—to reach out for and to communicate with the world.

Parents will learn very quickly which kind of handling is likely to be successful with their baby. This could be quiet speaking into his ear, or a gentle, firm touch on his belly. It could be a firm enclosing of his arms on his belly so that the startles that are set off by crying are interfered with and the cycles of crying will not keep building, or picking him up to contain and cuddle him, rocking or gently singing to him. Feeding him or allowing him to suck is almost a sure way to quiet any baby who is out of control. But if the calm is only temporary, the baby may be telling you to watch for some more important reason for the cries.

Very Sensitive Babies

Many babies are especially sensitive, what we call "hyper-sensitive"—to noise, to light, to maneuvers such as touch or massage, even to feedings. These babies deserve a gentle approach. Try only one thing at a time, as you test out what works for your baby. Speak quietly, don't look and feed at the same time, or rock and feed. Be sure you are in as peaceful an environment as possible. (See also *Small for Dates Babies* in Chapter 3.)

Active Babies

Because babies should not be put on their stomachs to sleep, this can make it more difficult for an active baby to quiet himself. On his back, he is at the mercy of sudden movements and startles. Each startle sets off a cry, another cycle of activity, and more crying. Very active babies have a tough time breaking out of this cycle—activity, startles, activity, startles—long enough to find hand-to-mouth comfort. On his belly, a baby's movements are limited and startles are contained. In this position, he can move around in bed, lifting his head from side to side, finally bringing an arm up to his head to suck on his thumb or fingers. But this position is safe only when he is awake, and you are there to turn him if he does begin to fall asleep.

Sleeping Position and SIDS

Today, parents are burdened with a new problem. We have learned that babies who sleep on their backs are less likely to suffer SIDS (Sudden Infant Death Syndrome). When babies can get bedclothes bunched up around their faces, they tend to rebreathe their own carbon dioxide exhalation. This makes them weak. They may then not be able to fight to clear their airways. And they may stop breathing. This can lead to SIDS. We now know that babies sleeping on their backs are more likely to be safe.

Though SIDS is a very rare occurrence, parents will want to take every precaution. Sheets, blankets, pillows, and stuffed animals can interfere with his breathing. A newborn has amazingly effective ways of freeing his airway, such as head turning and thrashing, coughing, pushing with his hands to try to sweep off any covering. But these don't always work. Loose or creeping wrappings that could reduce the oxygen to the baby should be removed from the crib. Any covering that interferes with easy air exchange can trap the carbon dioxide from his breathing and dangerously sedate a healthy baby. If this builds up, the oxygen decreases, he becomes dopey, and won't fight to clear his airway or to pick up his head and neck to free himself from whatever is blocking his breathing. Though babies are born with amazing defenses, the rare tragedy of SIDS makes us all careful.

Since it is also unsafe to try to contain the baby's startles by swaddling (a baby can wriggle down into his swaddling and suffocate), by pillows, or by tilting him on one side, if the baby is to be left alone, I have resorted to swaddling a fussy baby from the waist down. This way, his legs, at least, are not free to participate in the general startles that set off the cycling of startles and crying. This also leaves his hands free for him to find and suck on. Tilting the mattress slightly so that the movement of one arm is limited can certainly help eliminate startles. But this makes it easier for him to learn to push himself over onto his belly, making bedclothes and a soft mattress a danger. Parents of an active baby may be in for a challenging time. They will need to experiment with swaddling the legs and other ways described in the box earlier in this chapter on what to do when a baby cries.

Irritable Fussing at 3 Weeks ("Colic")

Between 3 and 12 weeks of age, most babies will develop a fussy, irritable period of crying, usually at the end of the day. Just as parents and siblings are getting weary, the baby becomes jumpier. He startles at small sounds. His movements are jerky. His face frowns. He holds his arms up tight, fists clenched. Legs are tightly thrusting. He acts as if his belly hurts and often spits up part of a recent feeding. Some babies regurgitate stomach contents into their esophagus, and the fussy irritability is blamed on "regurgitation" or "reflux." A pediatrician can prescribe medication to help an infant who has been diagnosed with gastroesophageal reflux. Most babies who cry during this period do not have true gastroesophageal reflux, but your pediatrician can evaluate your baby to be sure. In the absence of true reflux, medication has no established role.

Because this fussing is fairly universal, parents should know about this fussy period before it starts. By 3 weeks the increased feedings at the end of the day don't seem to satisfy the infant. His jumpiness and hypersensitivity predictably turn into fussing. Parents' awareness of this fussy period (I call it a "touchpoint") and its value for the infant may spare them unnecessary panic and anxiety. If they can see the fussing and crying as a necessary and even an organizing part of the baby's day, they won't have to feel so responsible. By predicting it and preparing them in advance, I have enabled many parents in my practice to cut the fussy period from 3 hours a day to 1 hour. We have not eliminated it, but we have made it manageable.

In the past, pediatricians called this fussy period "colic," because it was believed that the culprit was the digestive system—usually either gastroesophageal reflux or allergies to milk. Now we know that babies who cry at this age usually do not suffer from either condition. Instead, we have come to believe that this is a period during which the normal development of the infant's nervous system leads to most cases of this difficult-to-soothe crying. Yet all along, pediatricians have joined parents in an all-out effort to stop it each day. In the past we tried sedatives, and antispasmodics, but medications have no established role unless, as mentioned, an infant truly has gastroesophageal reflux, or another uncommon medical cause.

In the search for solutions, mothers have been urged to carry their babies and to nurse or feed them almost constantly. When this didn't work, mothers would call the doctor in desperation. Often they might call their own mothers. The grandmother might say, "Well, you were just like him." Fathers or friends might say, "If you'd put him on the right formula, he wouldn't fuss" or maybe "It's the way you handle him." The vulnerable new mother of course then felt like a failure. Mothers blamed themselves, and felt helpless. Every whimper from their infant felt like one more failure. Their tolerance for the child was often stretched. All of this makes it easier to understand why small babies are sometimes abused in this period. Fortunately we now understand more about this type of fussing.

Because I was curious about the common occurrence of end-of-the-day crying, and about its tendency to increase as parents' attempts to stop it became frantic, some years ago I did a study. I asked 80 healthy mothers to keep 24-hour records for the first 3 months. We learned a great deal. The mothers reported that their babies developed a predictably fussy period that began at the end of each day. It was a kind of cyclical crying, unlike pain or hunger. When the babies were picked up, handled, or fed either milk or water, the fussing subsided for a time. But the baby's jitteriness and frowning behavior did not subside. Any loud or sudden noise made them jump. A sudden change in light or position made them startle. The irritable crying started up again when they were put down. Even if they were carried, they were fussy and irritable. Nothing helped.

After this fussy period ended each evening, however, parents reported that their babies slept more soundly, ate more predictably, the length of time between feedings began to stretch out to 3 or 4 hours, and the babies seemed "ready" for the next 24 hours. With this information we began to see the fussy period as normal and even helpful. Understanding the value of the infant's fussing helped parents not to take each cry so personally.

Whenever a behavior is predictable and is as widespread as this, it tends to have an adaptive purpose. For those of us studying this fussing, it began to look like an organizing process—as if the baby were letting off steam from an over-loaded and immature nervous system at the end of the day. An immature nervous system can take in and utilize stimuli all through the day, but it overloads and may store up this overload, leading to shorter and shorter sleep and feeding periods. These short periods eventually build up to a blow-out at the end of the day. After this, the immature nervous system can reorganize for another 24 hours. As this pattern takes hold, the baby's cycle of sleeping and waking begins to be more regular. Mothers tell me that they have learned that the predictable end-of-the-day fussing means their in-fants won't need such irregular or frequent feedings. They eat only every 3 to 4 hours. They eat better at those times and sleep better in between. Their play is more advanced; they smile, and begin to vocalize. Being more alert for longer periods, they learn their mothers' rhythms and fa-thers' playful approaches.

I have come to believe that these difficult weeks serve a purpose. Not only does the end-of-the day fussing seem to set up more regular patterns of sleeping, waking, and feed-ing, but the baby also develops a new awareness of parents who have worked so intently during this period to comfort him. By 6 to 8 weeks, he will be able to distinguish his mother from his father, and both from a stranger. The learning that takes place during this period may well be related to a new organization of the nervous system—end-of-the-day fussing has been the difficult, but rewarding cost.

When I tell parents about this irritable period before it starts, they ask, "But how can we deal with it? Must we stand back and let him cry?"

I do not recommend just "letting him cry it out." I recommend that a parent try out all the maneuvers he can think of to find out whether the infant needs anything. (See box earlier in this chapter on "What To Do When a Baby Cries.") But try each only once. Pick him up and carry him to cut out the random, startling movements. Change him if he needs it. When he quiets down, offer him a feeding, but watch him to see whether he is really hungry. If not, don't overload his already full stomach. Then, resort to water feedings at regular intervals. The purpose of the water is to mobilize the air he will have cried down. "Colic" means a gassy intestine. And it's true that a crying baby gulps down air with each sobbing intake. Warm water every 10–15 minutes tends to produce opportunities to burp up bubbles. Nothing is as satisfactory to a parent as when the baby produces a loud, gassy bubble. A parent wants so badly to give her baby relief.

Don't do too much. Once you have assured yourself that your baby is not hungry, wet, or in pain, either resort to very

---

Handling Irritable Fussing

1. After checking to see whether he's hungry, wet, or in pain, put the baby to rest in a reclining chair or his bed for 10–15 minutes at a time.
2. Then, pick him up to burp him.
3. Feed him water. Some parents use "gripe water"* (a traditional home remedy) to help a baby get a bubble up, and to give him a chance to soothe himself by sucking.
4. Then, put him back down to let him fuss again for 5–10 minutes. You'll probably find, as I have, that he will fuss less if he's handled less. One to three hours of fussing is normal.

---

quiet, understimulating, soothing techniques or let him be. Gentle massage may help, if he's not too sensitive to touch at such a time. Try all the maneuvers outlined here, but when they don't work, stop! Too much handling or anxiety from parents can overload an infant's hypersensitive nervous system and will prolong this period of irritable crying.

---

* "Gripe water," used by previous generations and in many cultures today, is easily made up: 8 ounces water, 1 teaspoon of sugar, a tiny pinch of baking soda (too little baking soda is far better than even a little too much, which would be dangerous).

Watch the baby's face and his body. Learn his patterns. Is he quietly soothed after a burping? When you place him back in his reclining chair or on his bed, he will probably begin to look around, to frown slightly, to fuss quietly at first. Then he may build up to regular, cyclical crying. Bodily squirming, thrusting of arms and legs, facial frowns (but not as if in pain) are likely and expectable. If he quiets down when you pick him up to bubble him, you'll know this kind of fussing is not real pain.

Parents still worry about whether, if they let their baby cry for 10 minutes, they might miss a cry that truly needs attention. The baby will tell you. If he stops his fussing when you pick him up, if he quiets to look around, if he can suck the warm water and produce a bubble, if his body relaxes in your arms—you aren't likely to be missing a more serious reason. Even so, during this period he may start crying again as soon as you put him down. If, on the other hand, the crying gets worse and less predictable, it is always wise to seek advice from your pediatrician or nurse practitioner.

This necessary but trying period can be a "touchpoint," a time of learning for the baby and for the parent. I do not mean it to be a time to desert the baby's needs. If he cries more and more, he must be taken seriously. If this period increases in intensity and duration, I would want to look for other reasons—such as sensitivity to his milk, reflux of acid from his stomach into his esophagus, and other causes for such a distinct cry for help.

But this approach is well worth the try. Watch for the rewards ahead: After a bout of crying, the baby is ready to sleep and eat better. His sensitive, developing nervous system is reorganizing. Soon he will be able to smile, coo, and to recognize the difference between mothers, fathers, and others in his world.

4 to 6 Weeks

The baby's end-of-the-day crying may peak in this period, or shortly afterward. By this time, the baby's pediatrician or nurse practitioner should have seen the baby for a routine checkup. Despite any worries about the crying, if the baby is gaining weight and shows overall well-being, parents can feel reassured.

All the same, the crying that begins at 3 weeks can add stress to the developing parent-infant relationship. Many parents feel alone and frightened as a result. With enough support, however, parents can understand these important hurdles and feel equal to them.

When to Worry

There are a few important signs to watch for as you try to understand what your baby's cry is telling you.

An extremely piercing or high-pitched cry can be a cry of pain that means medical attention is needed. Normal crying at this age usually takes place during the late afternoon or early evening hours, at least three days a week. Crying that does not fit this pattern may have another meaning. This end-of-the-day crying usually lasts for not more than 3 hours. It usually begins at 3 or 4 weeks of age, peaks at about 8 weeks, and settles down at 3 or 4 months of age. If your baby's crying does not fit this pattern, or goes on to the same extent after 4 months of age, pediatric attention is needed.

Gastroesophageal Reflux. If your baby frequently regurgitates, vomits, and is losing weight, then he may in fact have gastroesophageal reflux. But be aware that 50% of all 2-month-olds will regurgitate at least twice a day. Infants with gastroesophageal reflux are a minority—less than 5% of infants under 3 months of age with "colic." Usually they have other symptoms too—choking, gagging, irritability, periods when breathing stops, hiccuping, feeding refusal (turning their heads away and arching, even when hungry), and weight loss, among others. These symptoms need to be assessed by a pediatrician.

(continued on next page)

When to Worry

(continued from previous page)

Milk Allergies.   Infants with milk allergies, also much less common than once thought (about 10% of infants under 3 months with "colic"), will sometimes have vomiting, diarrhea (at times with blood), and sometimes a family history of asthma or eczema. But there are plenty of milk substitutes that your child's pediatrician can help you decide to try.

Some Other Causes of Crying.   Very rarely, an infant this age can have a more serious reason such as heart disease or a migraine headache, two conditions leading to crying that is less likely to quiet when an infant is picked up and held. An infant with migraine headaches, though, usually has close relatives with a history of migraines. Persistent, difficult-to-soothe crying can also be a result of drugs to which the infant was exposed as a fetus in the uterus, or, on rare occasion, to drugs that a mother takes that can pass into breast milk. Finally, an infant this age who is being physically mistreated may also cry inconsolably. Many parents will worry about losing control when their crying baby can't be soothed. During this difficult period, parents and infants are more at risk. If your baby's crying seems to be more than you can bear, be sure to seek support from your pediatrician, nurse practitioner, or other healthcare professional. (See also *Resources for Parents.*)

Postpartum Depression

Postpartum depression afflicts roughly 10% of women during the first 12 months after delivery. It used to be thought that depressed mothers caused their infants' fussiness. Now, though, there is evidence that a fussy baby can actually increase a mother's risk for postpartum depression.

A mother who is faced with an infant's uncontrollable crying is bound to feel depressed and helpless. She is likely to try everything, and to overstimulate the baby, which will only make matters worse. She may feel that the baby's fussing is her "fault," and yet, she doesn't have a solution. A mother with postpartum depression, which may be full-blown just 6 weeks after delivery, worries that she does not love her baby or that she has not cared for him adequately. She may feel disconnected from her baby, and unable to enjoy him. It is easy to see how a fussy baby who is unresponsive to a mother's soothing might reinforce such feelings. Often a mother with postpartum depression may take her infant's cry as a criticism, or even a rejection.

Women with postpartum depression often do not recognize the signs, nor do their husbands and other family members. A father may feel desperate and ambivalent. With postpartum depression, it may be hard for a family to reach out for help. Yet if detected promptly, treatment of postpartum depression by a mental health professional can make a big difference—for the mother, and the baby.

Time-out for New Mothers

Whether a new mother has postpartum depression or not, she needs time out for herself through these difficult days of the infant's fussiness. Support from family, friends, pediatrician, or nurse is critical.

Our culture gives new parents less support than many others do. In Japan, in the Goto Islands off the coast of Nagasaki, a new mother returns to her own parents' household. There she is wrapped up on a futon, her baby at her side. Her parents, her in-laws, her aunts, and grandparents gather to take care of her for the whole first month. In that period she is helped to the bathroom, fed with chopsticks by her own mother, and massaged and treated like a baby herself. She is even spoken to in a high-pitched voice (as if she were a baby), and she responds in a high-pitched voice. Her only job is to feed and care for her new baby. Doctors in these islands tell me that there is no postpartum depression. After a month, the mother is expected to return to her home to care for her baby, and to help her husband tend his nets and clean his fish, for this is a fishing culture.

For parents everywhere, I long for at least some of the support and respect that parents in the Goto Islands are offered for the new job of parenting. I wish that families and medical providers in this country could offer parents reliable supportive care as they go through this important life adjustment.

An Infant Learns to Soothe Himself

As the infant grows, a major task for parents is to help the baby "learn" to comfort himself. I am always happy to see an infant who has already learned ways to comfort himself by 4–6 weeks—with his thumb or with a pacifier, or by finding a position in bed that comforts him. When we see a baby at Children's Hospital in Boston who sucks his thumb to comfort himself, we know that baby has developed inner resources to which he can turn when he's lonely or distressed.

I learn a great deal about a baby when I can watch him comfort himself. He wriggles around his crib, searching as if he knows that he must figure it out for himself, or he may lose control and be at the mercy of crying and startling. Self-soothing is the first step toward independence and a very early experience of success.

I have always urged parents to admire and to treasure a baby's ability to comfort himself. A pacifier can also be used to help the baby control his fussing so he can direct attention outward and learn about his world. I recommend an object to suck for all babies. (Of course, it must be unbreakable, too big to swallow, and nontoxic.) And of course, it can be the mother's breast or the baby's thumb, even as he is held in a parent's comforting arms. But, if the baby demands a mother's breasts too often, she is likely to wear out. Her breasts need to cycle: discharge, rest, discharge, with restful intervals for recovery and milk production. By 6 weeks, I like to see babies begin to cycle toward 3-hour periods for feeding and wakefulness. As we saw earlier, the fussy time at the end of the day seems to organize these cycles. They become more predictable, with more restful periods between feedings.

If a baby has not learned to comfort himself, I would try to encourage this during the day. At night, it is already becoming important for him to find his own self-comforting pattern when he rouses from deep sleep. So, work on it in the daytime. Help him find his fist or fingers, so that he can set up a pattern for sucking. A small infant's ability to comfort himself is valued differently from one culture to another. The kinds of self-comforting activities that are accepted can vary too. In mainstream American culture, the infant's thumb or pacifier are now widely accepted.

Sometimes patterns from our own past interfere with how we deal with crying and ways of self-comforting. With our first baby, I was eager for her to learn a self-comforting pattern. She was an easy baby, slept soundly, and waked for feedings in a predictable way. She started early to suck on her third and fourth fingers—an unusual pattern. She sucked vigorously and loudly, and obviously got a great deal of pleasure out of her finger-sucking. Yet I found myself pulling her fingers out of her mouth, as if I were trying to stop her. My wife pointed out that I wouldn't recommend that a parent try to stop finger-sucking in a new baby. When my own mother came to visit she noticed the sucking and said, "Isn't that amazing! Your baby sucks the same two fingers you did when you were a baby. I tried to pull them out of your mouth all the time." I then realized that my battle against her sucking came from a "ghost" in my own nursery.

Our patterns from our own past certainly dominate our behavior. As soon as I became aware of why I was so resistant, I could stop interfering. Recognizing our own "ghosts" can help us change our behavior toward our children. Our own childhood experiences of being nurtured are so critical to our ability to nurture. We bring both the good and the bad to our approaches and attitudes as parents.

8 Weeks

The fussing and crying at the end of the day may reach a peak as late as 8 weeks, and then begin to diminish. The reward for getting through the first stressful weeks, as the baby struggles to soothe and organize himself, is around the corner! If you are willing to stand quietly over the baby, talking to him, you may be greeted with a smile or coo. The crying and fussing have begun to give way to a baby who seems easier to know, and ready to play—an exciting touchpoint for parents and child.

Fussy crying spurts may no longer be restricted to the end of the day. They may occur unexpectedly, but be shorter and less frightening. They often now will seem to have a clear purpose. By now, an infant may have learned to call out to a parent with a whimper. If that doesn't work to get you to him, he'll either turn to soothing himself, or cry louder, more insistently. It's almost as if he were already learning the power of his cry—a way of getting you to feed him, change him, or just talk to him. He is already beginning to show that he needs periods of play with you.

In the morning and during most of the day, these demanding cries are easy to respond to. Some parents tell me that they even like to be called over. It makes them feel that they are necessary and the baby already knows it. But, toward the end of a busy day, when parents are tired, it's not always fun. Parents say they can even feel "manipulated" by such demanding cries. "And he's so little. What will he be like when he's older? I don't want to spoil him by going to him whenever he lets out a squeak."

New Rewards

Of course, it's important to respond. And the delighted greeting that you get back from your baby can be so rewarding. No one needs to be concerned that responding will spoil a baby this age. It is likely to do just the opposite. When you can give a 2-month-old baby what he needs in the way of a social response, he is much more likely to be a happy, contented baby. He will wiggle and squiggle whenever you show up and lean over him. He will know that you are there for him. Later, he will be ready to entertain himself when you can't.

At about this time, the wonderful reward of a smile from the baby begins to appear more regularly, and with a new certainty that he really means it. By 8 weeks of age, his smile seems to be voluntary and he can produce it more often, and may even be able to bring it out when he wants to. What a sure way to let his parents know he is doing well in their hands!

As the baby learns to use his whole face to express himself, parents become more aware of his ability to communicate with them. Each smile makes it more likely that parents will search for yet more ways to bring out another smile.

Parents have been learning how to handle the baby's crying episodes. Now they have begun to expect to have fun communicating with him too! The first real sign of a baby's cognitive development is his new ability to tell the difference between mother and father. (See box on page 45.) It is also a sign that infant and parents are on track with each other. Parents who must be away all day often say, "Will he know me?" The answer is yes.

Later during this period, at about 3 months of age, parents are able to imitate their baby's facial expressions in a way that makes it likely that he will respond with a smile. Their soft voices help them create a loving envelope around themselves and the baby. Then, their smiling behavior brings out a more and more reliable smile from the baby. Daniel Stern, a child psychiatrist and author, calls this phase "games" of interaction. A mother smiles, the baby smiles, the mother smiles, her baby responds—this goes back and forth in a rhythmic action three to four times. Meanwhile, every part of the baby's body is responding. His fingers, his toes, his legs, his arms, his face are all smiling and withdrawing the smile three to four times a minute. What parent wouldn't be ready to play such a game?

The more babies are smiled at, the more likely they are to smile frequently and in response to their parents' bids. A new, passionate parent is bound to smile more when the baby smiles. Such parents will feel "I'm really doing a great job!" They will feel successful and ready to search for other ways to react to him.

An Experiment

This is a way to see how much your baby has been learning during this period of disorganization and reorganization.

- Start with the mother and baby alone in a room.
- Prop the baby in a baby chair at a 45 degree angle.
- While doing this, avoid looking at him.
- Then sit down quietly in front of him, and talk to him.
- Watch his arms, legs, and facial expressions as you talk to him.
- When he smiles or goos at you, respond quietly in imitation. See whether he won't "talk" back and forth with his eyes, face, arms, hands, legs, and feet. Every part of him will recognize you with smooth movements. Three to four times every minute his fingers and toes will reach out and then settle back.
- Now ask the father to sit in front of the baby.
- Watch the baby's face light up. His eyebrows will lift. His eyes will sparkle. His feet and hands will jerk out to him, as if anticipating his father's kind of play.
- Watch the baby as his father starts poking and joking with him. Some fathers poke, some tickle, some play in other ways.
- Every part of the baby's body will be "up," anticipating the unique way his father approaches him.
- There may be many variations in parents' styles, but the baby will have learned the difference between each of *his* parents, and will already respond to each differently.

Recognizing Cries

By 8–10 weeks parents can recognize different kinds of crying more easily. The distinctions we saw earlier have grown clearer. By now, times for sleeping, waking, and feeding are starting to become slightly more predictable. The family can begin to imagine settling into a routine. This, too, makes it easier for parents to understand the meaning of a cry—too long since the last feeding or nap, too long awake without a chance to play. Parents now feel that they have begun to get to know their baby, and what will make their baby cry.

Boredom is a fussy, whimpering cry. His head will search for his fist or for the pacifier. He will stop when you lean over him or even when you talk to him from a distance.

Fatigue occurs at the end of a day, or after being exposed to a lot of excitement and stimulation. The cry is like the colicky, rhythmic cry at the end of the day. Soothe him, calm him, but don't give him too much more stimulation.

Hunger is accompanied by rooting and searching for something to suck on. When you feed him, it's obvious that this was what he needed. Watch how intently he focuses on the bottle or breast, or how his eyes lid down with pleasure and satisfaction.

Pain stands out at this age. You will have gotten used to his other cries. This one will startle you with its piercing, unrelenting quality. His face will be screwed into a tight knot. He will look at you with penetrating, beseeching eyes. He may bring his arms and legs up to his body in a tight ball, as if to protect himself. Or he may arch his back. Your heart will race, your lungs will be unable to fill up with air. You will feel desperate. His crying seems to go on forever, and may begin to sound less forceful as he tires. But nothing seems to give him relief for long. If by poking around gently you can't find the reason, it is time to call for help.

By this age, you and your baby will have learned so much about each other. Look back to the early days when you knew so much less. Every cry seemed the same—demanding something from you. A test. You didn't know what it might be. You tried everything, and it all seemed to make the crying worse. He escalated in his cries, instead of being comforted.

Now, with a few months of experience and learning, you feel you know the difference in his cries. Crying is still demanding, but your reactions are much more under control than they were. You can pick him up to cuddle him. You can sit and rock him. You can give him his thumb or a pacifier to see whether sucking will help. You can even croon to him or lean over to talk to him. You feel the miracle of being his parent. A kind of self-confidence is building up. Enjoy it, feel pride in all the learning that has gone into it—yours and his.

Maybe even the "colic" *has* served a purpose. You know now that you aren't likely to confuse it with real pain.

4 Months

Crying and Clear Communication

By now, the crying period at the end of the day has gone. (If it hasn't, then surely it is time to ask your child's health-care provider to evaluate your infant for other possible causes.) Cries of hunger, discomfort, boredom, and for attention are distinguishable. Routines are set, and feedings are usually predictable. If they are still happening too often, or their timing seems irregular, maybe you can let the baby fuss a bit before you go to him—to see whether he can fall back on his own resources. If he can't yet, it is time for you to help him begin to learn. He should be on a 3- to 4-hour cycle of eating, sleeping, and playing. By now, he should be able (1) to find his own fist; (2) to squirm around in bed to get into a comfortable position; (3) to accept his pacifier and to reach up with both hands to hold it lovingly; and (4) to enjoy a "reaching toy" over his bed to play with, or a visual mobile to look at. He won't do this for long, but long enough to let his parents know that he has new ways of entertaining himself—a major step in his development toward independence. And (5) he should be able to let you know when none of these works for him. His messages are clear. So are yours. You both feel you know each other.

Nighttime Cries

At night, the baby's cries are still piercingly demanding. But soon when he comes up to a semi-awake state every 3 to 4 hours, he may learn to scrabble around in bed to get himself back to sleep. In that case, he may be able to stretch out to sleeping for an 8- or 9-hour stretch. But he may not. At 4 months, many babies have not yet learned to put themselves back to sleep after the initial light sleep rousing that occurs every 3–4 hours. When the baby cries out, most parents feel that they must respond: with feedings, rocking and singing, a pacifier for soothing. They are looking for anything that works so "we can go back to sleep." Sleep-deprived adults are desperate. They can feel pushed to the edge by the child's crying and their own exhaustion. Fortunately, most parents restrain their out-of-control feelings and seek help. (See *Resources for Parents.*)

At this point, parents need to leave the baby in his bed, and help him learn to get himself back down to sleep. But the decision to begin to turn the job of getting to sleep over to the baby is not easy. The fussy, demanding cry that a baby of this age can muster makes parents feel they must (1) offer a feeding, (2) take the baby into bed with them, or (3) do anything out of sheer desperation.

Since it is hard to think about solutions during a sleepless night, every parent needs to pull back and reevaluate the situation—during the day. If the nighttime crying occurs only after special events, such as an exciting day, maybe it's the baby's way of letting off stored-up steam. If he wakes when he's lost his thumb or his pacifier, teach him gently how to find it. You may have to attach his pacifier to his sleeve so he can find it himself (but attach it loosely to avoid cutting off his circulation, and use a length short enough that it can't wrap around his neck, or any other part of his body). Since he must sleep on his back, he may not be able to cut out his upsetting startles. It may help to swaddle him from the waist down. Do this carefully so that there will be no loose covers into which he could creep and suffocate—especially if he is active at night.

Teach him how to calm himself down—not by letting him "cry it out" but by gently and firmly soothing him back down to sleep. You may feel so roused and angry that you transmit these feelings to him, but he needs to learn by modeling on your calm. Try to sit by his bed in a rocking chair to pat and soothe him: "You can do it. You can do it." While you're whispering this to him, you can also reassure yourself that you too can pull through these draining nighttime episodes.

The Beginning of Curiosity

Now, there's a new cry in the offing. At 4 to 5 months, there is a burst in awareness on the baby's part, a touchpoint. He begins to be much more inquisitive about the sights and sounds around him. But each touchpoint has its cost. The 4-month-old wants to look and listen to everything that goes on, and loses interest in the breast or bottle. His ability to reach out and play with toys now increases his interest in exploring these objects. He mouths them, he feels out every part with his fingers. As he finds something to feel, or to see, or to listen to, his face brightens up. He starts exploring. After three or four tries, he is bored. He whimpers. Or if he drops his toy, he whimpers. "Help me!" it says to a nearby parent. Restoring the toy to him may help once or twice, but soon it is apparent he's just bored with that toy. Another one helps briefly. Then, he starts fussing and tossing his head from side to side. It seems that nothing will help.

A frustrated but wise parent will pick him up to cuddle or carry. After a short time, put him in his crib to cool off. Fussing at first, he may drop off to a short nap. Afterward, he'll be ready again for more exploration. But probably nothing will satisfy him for long. He is on a roll toward a new level of exploration, play, and adjustment. Feeding, sleeping, old routines—all are affected. Does this new kind of crying mean he is bored, demanding, fatigued, or dissatisfied with himself? All of the above. Even an attentive parent will have to let him work it out.

The First Layer of Stranger Awareness

When I see a baby in my office at this age, the baby is likely to smile and chortle at me across my desk. But when he is placed on my examining table to be undressed, his face sobers and his body tenses. He is warning us that he is aware of the strangeness of the surroundings. His bodily behavior lets me know that he is very sensitive to anything new. If I lean over to look and talk to him at this point, he is bound to dissolve in loud, protesting cries. If I add my voice to try to comfort him, his cries will increase. If I try to pick him up to cuddle him, he'll protest even more.

This is an early sign of "stranger awareness." (Usually, it becomes full-blown by 8 months.) He does not want to be handled in a strange situation by a stranger. Grandparents beware. When I first realized this, I began to place his parent right next to me and the baby, so that he did not have to look at me as I examined him. It worked. In this way an infant will let me prod and poke, listen to his heart and lungs, even examine his ears and throat, as long as all he can see is his parent.

Fun and Games

Which parent is most likely to make a baby laugh? His father! Our research has shown that babies respond differently to mothers, fathers, and others. They have a different set of responses for each of the important adults. As you may have noticed if you tried the experiment earlier in this chapter, a mother is likely to draw out quiet, smooth movements of the baby's arms, legs, fingers, and toes and gentle facial brightening with a smile. When his father looms in sight, everything about him changes. His face goes up, his eyebrows, eyelids, mouth, head all go up to greet him. His fingers, toes, arms, and legs reach out toward his father, jerkily. He is more likely to laugh than to smile. To chortle rather than coo. Every part of his body is ready to be poked and he is primed to play. He has already learned that each parent is different, and he is trying to anticipate these differences by differences in his own behavior. He knows them as individuals and shows it.

As the baby's ability to use his facial muscles in a smile increases, his smile becomes more and more available and exciting to those around him. He can attract people. He can hold onto them. He begins to feel a sense of power. By 4 to 5 months, as his interest in the world around him enlarges, he will often let out a cry or a vocal bid for attention. When he brings his target close, his smile widens. All of his face is involved in this effort. He is recognizing that his smile has power! He may even chortle. Laughing or chortles are most likely to follow something that is unexpected.

In the next few months, games like peek-a-boo—with a surprise attached—will become exciting to a 6- to 8-month-old baby. When the game is set up, and the surprise comes, he will laugh out loud; his laughter is contagious. After a laugh, a parent will try to tickle him to get another laugh. The laughing and the peek-a-boo surprise game go on until the baby tires and says with his eyes and his head turning away, "I've had enough!"

Smiling and laughter are developed over the child's infancy and childhood as ways of bringing important people to them. In the little games that follow, both baby and adult feel the glow of a reliable and rewarding communication system!

If a 6-month-old baby does not respond to an adult or to another child with these smiles or wiggles or coos, I'd be concerned about whether that child was depressed or withdrawn, or delayed in his social development or communication skills. It may be a signal that an evaluation by a mental health professional who understands babies might be needed.

Cooing

When, in our research, a baby is placed in a baby chair, the parent leans over him to start off an interaction. In a 3-minute period, they communicate back and forth in rhythmic behaviors. Smile–smile, coo–coo. The baby gurgles, reaches out with arms and legs, gaily lets the parent know, "You are here with me, and we are communicating!"

The baby is able to maintain control over his startles, and react in a series of imitations, during such "games." Cooing is part of these predictable games. Though he reacts differently to a mother, or to a father, or to another in these games, the sounds he makes are predictable and prolonged. For at least three or four coos, a mother usually stays in her seat, cooing back and interacting. With his father, the cooing is likely to escalate into a squeal by the third or fourth. Soon the father will be leaning forward, edging out of his seat to poke or tease the baby to a peak of excitement. A mother is likely to be gently, quietly soothing and content with the baby's soft coos.

By 6 to 7 months, the cooing is beginning to take shape into a murmured "mum–mum–mum" or even a "da–da–da." It has always been interesting to me that fathers were assigned the excited, giddy "da–da." Babies chortle, squirm, and work hard as they express these sounds. With the "mum–mum" they are likely to be trying to quiet and soothe themselves. Are they already "saying" what they've learned to expect with these early "words"? Or do parents teach the "da–da" and "mum–mum" sounds to help babies tell the difference between parents' roles? At 6 or 7 months, the meaning of these sounds has not yet been mastered. But they already are part of the games that parents will play with their babies.

7 to 8 Months

A "Help Me" Cry

At 6 months, and unable yet either to support himself with his arms or to roll down and over, a baby will sit like a lump in a slumped-over position. His chin is on his chest, his fat stomach protruding. He tries to straighten up, but after a brief try, his head slumps toward his belly again. If you appear, he straightens up to look at you with accusing, longing eyes: "Why did you put me in this position? I can't even use my new reaching. All I can do is slump, and I'm helpless." He groans, he complains, and finally he wails as if to say "Help me!" The cry is sharp, and demanding. Any parent is likely to get the message, "Either pick me up, or lay me down so I can roll to where I want to go. Or, prop me better in a reclining position so I can reach for toys and keep myself amused. But don't desert me."

At the same time, this desire to get out of a passively dependent situation drives a baby to learn how to use his body. In the next month, he is likely to be able to roll down to a flattened position, to roll over onto his belly, and to creep—all in one elegant, continuous movement. A watching parent may not realize it, but he's on his way to independence. The frustrated cry and whimper may precede this new skill, but they won't need to last long. He will use his frustration to find a solution for himself.

Meanwhile, as reaching has been perfected, he may cry out with another kind of frustration. He wants to pick up small objects on the floor as he crawls. He begins by clasping his whole hand to pick it up. But that doesn't work. By 7 or 8 months, he works, works, works, reaching out for an object, trying to handle it. He knocks it off the table. He *looks down* to get it. We call this "object permanence"—he knows the object still exists even when it has disappeared! He can't reach it, so he cries out "Help me!" A willing parent will be at the mercy of these cries. If you hand the object to him, he turns it over, bangs it, and clumsily drops it again. Knowing you are there and are ready to play his game, he cries out again—and again—and again. Parents wonder, "Should we go get it over and over?" Sure, if you want to be involved in his game of "go fetch." But as he tries to reach objects himself, he will surely learn to become more agile—eventually.

Turning Cries of Frustration into Learning

The baby's frustration at not being able to do what he wants can be a powerful force for learning. Watch him when you put him to bed at night. He will likely turn over and crawl. He is also likely to put his hand up to look at it in the light, to admire it, and to work his fingers as if he were trying to picture how to make them work better. In fact, his crying protests at being put to bed may suddenly stop as he turns to this important honing of his skills. When we put one of our own children to bed at this age, we expected he'd cry out in protest, despite all of our soothing bedtime rituals—rocking, singing softly, reading. But when the protests stopped so suddenly, we rushed in to see whether he might have choked—or smothered—or fulfilled any of our fears. He was just practicing his new tricks, and we felt a bit absurd.

Silence as a Danger Signal

As the desire to creep and even to crawl builds up, another cry appears. Now he can get into spaces where he gets stuck. He may cry out in helplessness. You must go to him to help him. He may even be in danger, but cannot be relied upon to warn you that he's in danger. His new mobility demands that a parent thoroughly check the safety of the area where the baby is left. He may be so interested in his new ability to get around, turn over, seek new surfaces and objects to explore that silence can be a more serious warning than protesting cries.

As he becomes more skilled in grasping and exploring with his fingers, silence may hide another danger. Quietly and contentedly, he will pick up and mouth everything he can find—including small objects he can choke on, sharp ones that can damage his insides, and dangerous household poisons. Get down on your hands and knees; check out what he might find everywhere in the house. When you can hear him crawling about, with protests and occasional cries of determination, you can be more certain of his whereabouts and safety. Silence can be warning you, "I'm getting into trouble."

Stranger Anxiety

At about the age of 8 months, full-blown stranger anxiety appears. You take the baby to Grandma's. Your sister is there. Everyone rushes to greet you—and him. Everyone wants you to hand him over, but wisely you resist: "Let him get used to you first while I hold him. These days he doesn't like to be handed from person to person." Meanwhile, he's redoubled his clinging to you. You are too busy talking to notice it. You know he knows these relatives. But you begin to be aware of his rigid body, his tight clasp on your clothes, and his frozen face—staring rather desperately at your mother and sister. All of a sudden, someone moves or speaks or reaches out to him. He begins to wail. Screaming, hiding his face, he pulls at you frantically. Everyone rushes over to help you. This only makes him scream more loudly. He barely catches his breath. Your family asks, "What in the world is this?" You look at the floor for a hole to sink into.

Unfortunately, "this" represents an expectable developmental process that appears at 8 months. Parents are not surprised if the baby wails and withdraws when there is indeed a stranger present. "But these are familiar, dear people. My own sister seems to be frightening to him. My mother, who sits with him so often, suddenly terrifies him. What in the world is happening?"

What has happened can be explained, and is predictable. A new burst in cognitive development has brought on the ability to make comparisons, and fine differentiations. Now he is struck with the subtle differences between his father and his father's brother, his mother and his mother's sister. Grandparents who have been part of the baby's life will now need to be patient, and wait until he can look them over. The baby must get used to these new differences he is mastering. His frightened response to the differences he now sees between familiar relatives shows how he is working to understand important cues in his world. This period may last only a few weeks or a month, but it is an important one: The baby is developing his ability to make ever finer distinctions.

As a pediatrician, I learned never to look a baby this age in the face when I first meet him. If I do, I can expect immediate retreat behind loud wails and crying. Of course, no new or eager person should take a baby this age from a parent. These cries are defenses against being overwhelmed by new, exciting, but intrusive experiences. The protest represents the amazing and passionate learning that is going on at this age. Protecting the baby becomes a parent's first job. A parent can warn relatives and friends ahead of time: "Don't try to take him from me or look him right in the face. At this age, he is wary of anyone but us." If the "stranger's" presence alone brings on the crying anyway, take the child aside to cuddle and croon over him in a familiar way. Give him a chance to recover.

When Wailing Means "I Missed You"

Infants in childcare seem to handle this stage differently. They learn to accept caregivers other than their parents, without the same need to retreat and to protest. However, they often fall apart and cry at the end of the day when their parents arrive to pick them up. This kind of crying may also come from a baby's new ability to tell parent and stranger apart, and from his saved-up longing for his parent. Unfortunately, some childcare workers may comment: "He never does that to me." Devastated, a parent feels even more shut out by the baby's protests. But a parent who understands what is happening needn't feel hurt. Pick the baby up to hug him, to cuddle him, to croon to him. He's missed you, and wants you to know it.

Whenever you appear after an absence, that kind of crying may become expectable. Understand it as your baby's attempt to reunite with you—intensely, passionately. Introduce a "lovey," a cuddly object or piece of blanket for him to use as a substitute for you when you are away. This lovey will also be a way of encouraging the baby to comfort himself. The lovey makes possible a form of self-soothing, which helps him develop self-control. Some parents wonder, "But will he ever give it up?" He will, when he's ready to become more independent. Meanwhile, his thumb and his lovey are such wonderful companions for him on this exciting road to independence.

10 Months

Crying Out for Limits

As the baby begins to explore on his own, handling things with his increasingly precise grasp, a parent needs to be more aware than ever of the dangers in the house, and everywhere the baby spends time. At the same time, the baby becomes aware that his explorations can make everyone jumpy! He will become fascinated with these new ways of engaging his parents' attention. He crawls up to the stove or the forbidden TV set. He looks around to be sure a parent is nearby and ready to say "DON'T TOUCH." If there is no parent available, he is likely to cry out, as if *imitating* his own crying. He already knows that this will bring them to him. When they arrive, he is likely to scramble with an increasingly rapid crawl, enticing parents to chase after him.

Cries of Protest, Cries of Relief

"No" isn't enough. The child knows that already. He is waiting for a more active decision—being picked up, removed, even closed away from the exciting, forbidden object. His loud protests contain a trace of relief. He may be learning to mix "yes" and "no" in these protests. If you, as a parent, listen for it, you will hear: "Thank goodness someone knows how to stop me." Thank goodness someone cares enough!

New Skills and a New Cry for Help

At night, the baby may practice his new ability to pull up on the railing and stand at the side of his crib, hanging on. He will stand there as often as every 3 to 4 hours, calling out and crying as if he can't get back down. Parents tell me: "He needs me! He can't find his own way back down." Innocently, I ask, "Can he get up and down by himself in the daytime?" "Of course!" "Isn't it interesting that he won't try it for himself at night?" I observe. Parents protest, "But he may not even be fully awake." They are probably right. The baby's drive to practice newly learned skills surfaces each time he comes up to light sleep. If you want a baby to learn to handle this and get himself back down, you may have to urge him to see that he can do it by himself. By this I don't mean just leaving him there to scream. If you go to him and just give him a gentle shove so that he folds in the middle, he'll discover that he can do it for himself. He can also learn to put himself back to sleep after every waking from light sleep. Parents can sit beside the crib to comfort him. Say quietly over and over, "You can do it yourself. You can do it yourself."

Often, parents call me a week later to tell me that he has learned that he can come to a light sleep, wake up and start moving around, stand up but then get himself back down. The sleep pattern has been saved!

A Toddler's Cries

Frustrated Crying

With walking, and his new independence, a toddler may also begin to act more dependent. He is likely to collapse in screams at the end of the day. He may dissolve into crying fits before each meal, each nap. It is as if he were saying, "This reaching out for independence—walking, going around the corner from you, learning to tease you to react—is costing me a lot. One of the only ways I can deal with it is to fall apart."

The desperate wailing is heartbreaking. It can be understandable at times—before a nap, or when he's falling apart at the end of the day. The toddler may also wail when confronted with any change—for example, a new person, a new place, a sudden noise, or even when his other parent comes in. "He seems so fragile. Is he sick or is something wrong with him?" Never ignore signs of illness or pain. But the crying may be just a sign of the intensity of his new life. He is learning to balance on his feet, even to dare to let go with his hands. He must leave the comfort of his mother's side or his father's arms in order to go exploring. He'll certainly fall down and wobble about. The cries can come from the frustration of wanting so much to succeed at walking. When he falls down on his soft bottom, he is likely to let out a cry of frustration, not pain.

No Longer a Baby

When you pick him up to comfort him, he may fall apart even more. In this protesting behavior is the message, "Put me down and let me work it out myself." That's a tough, new message for parents.

When the toddler staggers into the next room, he may suddenly cry out as if in pain. You rush to his side and he seems comforted to see you. But he won't let you pick him up, or even stay in his sight. You may have even figured out that his cry was one of fear at being alone in a dark room or a forbidden kitchen. He certainly needs your comfort—but only briefly. He is striving to balance this with another goal: independent exploration.

As the toddler begins to explore his universe on his own, thanks to the amazing new ability to walk, he begins to feel the excitement of independence. But it carries a frightening cost. "Will Daddy be there if I disappear around the corner? Did he really get mad at me for climbing the stairs alone? If I touch the forbidden stove (to find out if it is really "HOT"), will he be angry for a long, long time?" This emotional cost is written on his face as he explores. He nearly always looks back to see whether a parent is watching as he sets off on his little adventures. If no one is watching, he may let out a loud, demanding cry.

But when Daddy comes around the corner, his face may be confusing to the toddler. He may look half angry, glaring, his mouth turned down. But his relief at finding the toddler unharmed may show too. When he holds out his hand to stop some dangerous move, of course the toddler doesn't want to be stopped! He wants to go on and on—

exploring and learning. So he falls in a heap on the floor, screaming and thrashing. If parents try to comfort him, it only gets worse. A parent may well join the screaming. "Be quiet! Stop that tantrum!" But such efforts will only make matters worse. (See *Temper Tantrums* in Chapter Three.)

At such moments, you are likely to feel unwanted by your child, even deserted. "Why do you cry out as if you need me, and then when I come in, you don't want me?" A toddler's crying out for help at almost every turn can become so grating and demanding that you can feel annoyed, even angry. You may feel like saying, "Be quiet! Either you need me or you don't, but you just confuse me with your crying!" Your confusion matches his. He wants so much to be independent, but he is frightened at the same time. He knows he is not quite ready for all the dangers and excitement that his walking and new skills have led him into.

This is truly a touchpoint, when a child's uncertain confidence about separating from you does not match his new ability to "get around" on his own. It won't last. He will become more comfortable with independence. But when that happens you then may have to face the fact that you have "lost" your baby—and you may find that it is your turn to cry.

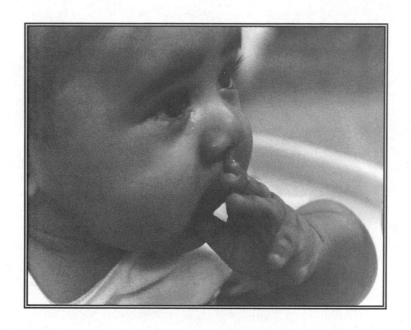

CHAPTER 3

The Messages in a Child's Cries

Attention-Getting

Even with a newborn, parents are likely to feel, "She cries just to get my attention!" A mild cry, which quiets as soon as you go to her, makes a parent feel "used." Angry, a parent may even walk away. Then, the cry can build up to a more demanding one, and a parent will have to come back and do something (such as picking her up, or feeding her). Perhaps it would be easier in the first place to lean over her, to engage her with coos and soft talk. But, in the back of a parent's mind is, "Am I spoiling her?" As she gets older and becomes more skilled at calling for your attention, there will be times when you will need to lean over her, to say, "You can manage yourself."

It is hard to imagine spoiling an infant, because it is so necessary for the parent to learn about her with each cry. But by 4 or 5 months, as we saw in Chapter Two, it is possible to leave her for brief periods to amuse herself. As she grows older, and her cries are easily recognized as "demanding" or "spoiled," limiting your responses may be a way of saying, "You can manage this yourself." I'd respond once, then when your response is not enough, turn it back to her to manage. A spoiled child is one who doesn't know how to impose limits on her own demands, and, by her behavior, asks for limits from you. If you watch her face after you've given her a firm reply, she may seem to relax and smile— almost in thanks, as if the limits from you were reassuring.

Crying in the second year, or even in the first year, that is aimed at parents and that has no obvious cause except to demand attention makes everyone wince. An anxious, unresourceful child who exhibits this kind of crying may be labeled as spoiled. Though the demanding crying is aimed at getting a response from adults, its very quality carries a message: "You can't satisfy me." A spoiled child is one who has never learned her own limits, never learned to entertain and comfort herself. She has lived in an overprotective or an overindulgent environment.

Some parents may try to do everything for a child. Perhaps there has been an earlier worry about the child—for example, prematurity, illness, the effect on the child of a family problem or a tragic event. Parents may feel that they have failed the child in some way. Other parents may be trying to make up for feeling that they'd been failed or short-changed as a child. In these situations, when the child must face another stress, even a small, everyday one, parents may rush in too soon. The child then misses out on facing the challenge for herself, facing her frustration and the need to try again. She will miss out on the all-important sense of "I did it *myself!*" This feeling is essential to her future self-image, her sense of her own competence. Without this, a child is often whiny and fussy and cries a lot.

The parent of a child like this needs to reconsider her approach. Maybe she isn't leaving enough up to the child. Without realizing it, she may not be allowing the child to discover her own abilities. Maybe she is unclear about the limits that this child needs to feel safe. For children like this I recommend these steps:

1. Set clear limits and present them with your confident belief that limits are a gift, not a punishment.
2. Let the child work to experience her own sense of achievement.
3. Offer, point out, and even insist on tasks (such as calming herself down, amusing herself when she is

bored) that will give a child the chance to experience this sense of achievement.

4. Encourage your child to find her own pride in her success. Instead of "I'm proud of you" substitute "Do you realize what you just did? Aren't you proud?" She can even be proud of overcoming her frustration!

5. Meanwhile, to prevent her from feeling as if you are deserting her, pick her up to love her at times in between episodes, when she is not demanding your attention. Then, both you and she can feel safer when you need to push her to "do it herself" at other times.

Breath-Holding

Breath-holding events are most likely to occur between 6 months and 5–6 years. In the second year, a toddler may hold her breath in the midst of a temper tantrum. She may hold it long enough to turn blue or she may faint. Frightening indeed! Parents may want to rush her to an emergency room or think it's necessary to give her mouth-to-mouth breathing. But before you can act, her breathing is likely to return to normal, and she will be alert again. These episodes when added to temper tantrums can make parents feel helpless and terrified. They may even feel driven to try to avoid temper tantrums at all costs—almost impossible in the second year. But the efforts to coddle a toddler may even add to her tantrums.

If these episodes occur at a peak of the child's frustration or anger, they are likely to be normal and nothing needs to be done. In fact, any tension and the short-lived hysteria they cause in parents can reinforce the tension in the child. A calm, reassuring approach may do most to help the child learn to handle these peaks of disintegration.

But if breath-holding occurs often, and doesn't seem to be triggered by tense events, frustration, transitions, or a parent's unwanted limits, the child's physician should be consulted. Involuntary breath-holding can look to parents like a seizure, and they will need to contact their physician. Young infants who stop breathing during sleep for more than fifteen seconds need to be roused by parents. If breathing does not begin with rousing, call 911 and begin CPR for infants (see American Heart Association CPR at www.amherst.edu).

But for most children, these events are a result of overwhelming anger or frustration that starts out first as a tantrum. The breath-holding occurs at the peak of the disorganized behavior, and if it causes the toddler to pass out, the breathing should resume right away. This kind of breath-holding passes too soon to cause any brain damage, which any parent fears. These frightening events are usually harmless and do not require any treatment. However, a parent who witnesses these events certainly deserves the advice of the child's physician.

Fear of Independence

In the second year a particular kind of crying arises from the child's struggle between dependence and independence. Every sudden change calls up this conflict. When you dress her to go out, or when you take off her coat as she comes in. When she goes to Grandma's or to school, to familiar and even beloved places, she is likely to become clinging, and will whimper about being torn away from you. You are likely to wonder why she is so fragile, so dependent all of a sudden. You thought she loved to be in new places, and certainly in familiar ones. Why does she fall apart at the idea of going out? She even cries and falls apart when you come to get her.

Why this new behavior? A toddler's conflict about becoming more independent is near the surface. Her urge to take any new step calls up her own feelings of vulnerability—"I'm so little." But watch her strut around when she wins a struggle or when she can conquer this indecision about her need to be independent. She will need her thumb and her lovey to face these challenges.

Nightmares and Fears

Nightmares and new fears begin to surface in 4- and 5-year-olds. Phobias (intense fears) about barking dogs or loud ambulances are coupled with fears that may seem unreasonable and "out of the blue." Nightmares are likely to be about monsters or witches, under the bed or in the closet. All of these are new and a surprise to child and parents. As the child dissolves in tears, parents will wonder, "What in the world brought this on?"

These fears and nightmares are predictable at this age. They do not necessarily mean that the child has been traumatized or frightened by an experience. They can come from a developmental process in the child. She is beginning to be aware of her own aggressive feelings. As they bubble to the surface, she is likely to yell at the top of her voice, to argue with every other classmate, to cheat to win, and to worry.

What does she worry about? Her "badness." Strong urges to try out "being bad" are enough to make a child feel scared—of herself! In the daytime, if she is about to be left alone, she may show unexpected fearfulness and vulnerability. When lightning strikes, or when a fire engine roars by, a child this age is likely to take it as a punishment—for wanting to try out "being bad." Her vulnerability shows up as a new fear or a phobia. She may refuse to walk by a house with a barking dog.

These fears may be kept under control in the daytime, but they will come out at night—when she is all alone. When she must be left, and must go to sleep, the fears come to the surface. Sobbing, and curled up in a ball, she wriggles under the covers. "Don't leave me! She'll come and get me!" "Who will?" "The witch!" "What witch?" "The one with the pointy teeth and the long claws." "You can't mean she's here in your room." "I do, I do! When you turn off the light, she'll come out."

Fears and Crying at Night

To help a child overcome nighttime fears, there are several steps that you can take:

1. Look under the bed with her.
2. Open the closet door and show her it's empty.
3. Cuddle her one more time to reassure her.
4. Don't ridicule her.
5. Sit by her bed to sing her a lullaby and to soothe her. Offer her "lovey" to comfort her.
6. Leave on a nightlight.
7. Ask yourself why she's suddenly so frightened.
8. Check at school or with her other caregivers to be sure there's been no trauma.
9. Watch for her aggressive bursts. Don't squelch her, but point out how hard she's working to handle herself.

(continued on next page)

Fears and Crying at Night

(continued from previous page)

Encourage her to play and to talk out these feelings during the day. Dolls, puppets, and action figures can help.

10. Let her model herself on you. How you handle your own aggression will help her to "learn" to handle her own feelings in safe ways. Perhaps you might say, "I felt like punching that lady who cut in front of me at the store, she was so mean. But I didn't. I just held it in, until I left. Then I yelled to myself to let off steam. Do you ever feel that way?" She may be able to respond. She may not. But her wide, observant eyes will let you know that she's taken it in.

11. Let up on pressure, but don't change the rules. You may have to choose your battles all over again. This is a time to expect rougher play, and to let some of this slip by. But when she's aggressive enough to scare herself, she'll need discipline more than ever: "I have to stop you when you do that. Every time you do it, I have to stop you until you can stop yourself." Discipline that is fair and familiar is reassuring at such a time.

12. Expect her fears and her nightmares to decrease as she learns to handle her "badness" (her aggressive feelings) more comfortably. Meanwhile, the fragility that goes with this learning process will cause unpredictable crying over a period of several months in this "growing up" period. (See *Touchpoints Three to Six,* listed in the *Books for Parents* section.)

Sadness

Depression can occur at any age. It sends a message, "I'm not getting what I need." When a baby is "not right," and just seems irritable and sad, it is time to look for underlying reasons. She may not eat right or sleep well. She may be awake, eyes open, staring into space. Or she may be fussy and unable to be comforted. You may notice apathy, easy fatigue, little interest in toys or things around her, or the reverse side of the coin—an irritable response to everything. These symptoms usually come with losses, separations, and perceived failures. They may also reflect her feelings of worthlessness. Or she may be suffering from a physical illness that needs to be identified and treated.

Helping a Sad Child

1. Hug her, rock her, sing to her often.
2. Talk to her and pay attention to her pleas. Watch her for cries, and share her sadness.
3. Try to understand what is underlying it. Listen. Talk with others who care for her.
4. Bolster her self-esteem at every turn.
5. Set aside special times for her alone, and talk about these times in between.
6. If her symptoms persist and you aren't able to help her, seek psychological evaluation.

Separations

When a child looks up at you, her thumb in her mouth, her eyes sad, her face drawn, her shoulders down, it is very difficult to leave her. Her cry at these moments has an emptiness and a kind of soft, wailing quality. She now knows, beforehand, how upset she'll be when you go. She knows how upset you'll be too. A parent can lose her determination. Not only the child's crying, but her resourcefulness in delaying the separation—thwarting her parents' efforts to dress her or to get her fed—can wear a parent down. One mother told me that her child would undress herself on the way to preschool. She'd arrive naked in order to delay this separation.

Handling Separations

1. Always prepare a child ahead of time—no matter how difficult it is to face her protest. "You'll be at your school while I'm at work. I'll be back at the end of the day, and we'll have supper and read together. I'll miss you, and I know you'll miss me."
2. Promise her a time when you'll return, one you can be sure to stick to.
3. When the wailing and resistance begin, hug her to help her into the car or bus, or at the door of the childcare center. Be sure to encourage her to use her thumb and her lovey to comfort herself. "You can squeeze your lovey hard and make her feel better."

(continued on next page)

Handling Separations

(continued from previous page)

4. Share her sadness with teachers or caregivers so someone whom she knows and trusts is ready to hold her.

5. Use her favorite teacher or caregiver to help her get comfortable and to engage her in an interesting task.

6. Stay a few minutes to help her with the transition, but be definite about leaving when you must. (In the beginning, though, I'd certainly stay until she's used to her new surroundings.) Your unvoiced distress about leaving her can make her feel that you don't really trust the caregivers you must leave her with—adding fear to her sadness.

7. When you do return, remind her of the promise you've kept ("Daddy always comes back"). Remind her of the cuddles and the story reading to come, the time together that you'd promised. You can even encourage her to use what she's learning for the next separation: "When I have to leave you tomorrow, you can remember how I always come back."

8. Admire her for being able to let you go. Tell her you know she worried about you, but everyone at school loves her too, and you'd never leave her longer than you had promised.

9. When you are together, try playing some games that help a child to remember that you are still somewhere even when you are not visible to her. Peek-a-boo, hide-and-seek, or hiding and finding an object are games that help a child practice holding on to her image of you even when you are not there.

Small for Dates Babies

Babies who weigh too little for their height at birth may be "small for gestational age" (SGA) or "small for dates." While they may be born to mothers who had had normal pregnancies, normal nutrition, and did not smoke or use drugs or alcohol, these babies often behave quite differently. They are a bit slower to rouse and to feed, and frown all the time. When picked up to cuddle, they get very tense. They pull up their arms and legs in a tight, worrisome position. All of these movements seem to be aimed at protecting themselves. These skinny, worried-looking babies often have a hypersensitive nervous system. If those who care for them speak in a soft, soothing voice, they can gradually adjust. Handle them gently and wait for them to relax before looking at them or rocking them. Look or handle or talk—one activity at a time—never all at once.

At 2–3 weeks of age, these babies begin to cry in a special way—often after difficult feedings, which parents attempt every 1–2 hours to help them "catch up" in weight. The cry is a high-pitched, piercing, demanding cry. When they are talked to, they are likely to turn their heads away. When a parent tries to comfort them, they spit up, have a bowel movement, or start to hiccup. Their faces can look angry and withdrawn. Parents may feel that these babies are saying, "You are not good for me." All this makes new parents feel like failures. If parents can be prepared ahead for this difficult crying and lack of responsiveness, they don't have to feel so rejected by their newborn.

This high-pitched, demanding crying can last 3–5 hours a day, from 2–3 weeks until 12–16 weeks of age. Swaddling helps. Carrying them next to one's body helps. Cutting down on other kinds of stimulation helps. These babies gradually outgrow their highly sensitive reactions as their central nervous systems mature. But they often remain sensitive and overreactive even throughout the first year. The early months with these babies are difficult for any parent.

For these babies, I advise as little extra stimulation as possible. Use quiet surroundings, carrying, swaddling, a soothing voice, gentle rocking, and soft singing. The high-pitched, demanding cry may be difficult to live with, but expect it whenever the baby cries. The usual gradations in crying and in bodily responses may not be present, and these babies can be very hard to read. Above all, be patient. The small for dates babies whom I've known in my practice have turned out to be engaging, intelligent, quickly responsive children later on, as their parents allowed them time to mature at their own pace.

Temper Tantrums

I have learned that a temper tantrum is a child's issue, not a parent's. We must leave it to her to settle: "Will I or won't I? Do I want or don't I?" What sets a tantrum off seems unimportant and unexpected to a parent. But it obviously has real meaning for the toddler. Underneath the 2-year-old's tantrum often lies the feeling of being torn between two opposite wishes, or between wanting independence and being scared of it.

Parents are bound to feel helpless when they are unable to control the child, and on the verge of losing control themselves. Child abuse can occur in the second year as a result of the feelings that these tantrums stir up in parents. When these tantrums occur in public places, as they are likely to do, parents feel exposed as "bad parents." Unable to help or to stop the insistent wailing and thrashing, they feel helpless, inadequate, even guilty. Every onlooker adds to this as they glare at the parent and the fallen-apart child. I have found that the surest way to end such an episode is to turn one's back on the scene. When you walk away (if she's safe) or stop reacting, the force of her tantrum is lost. You are saying, "You can handle this yourself."

Then, when it is over, return to pick her up and hug her, saying, "It feels terrible to get so upset." In this way, let her know you accept her as she is. You can even understand the inner confusion she is experiencing. In a way, you are also saying, "I wish I could help you, but I can't." And indeed, she will have to learn to make decisions herself rather than depending on a parent to make them for her. She is torn between one desire and its opposite, wants both, but can have only one. Parents are confused, because the child's choices don't seem important enough to lead to such explosions. Stepping back to let her settle herself is a little like encouraging her to soothe herself—for example, with a lovey, or her own thumb. When she discovers that she can master these feelings, she will feel less at their mercy.

By the time a child is 2 years old, she begins to realize how powerful her demands can be. Her temper tantrums are even more dramatic. Coupled with the feeling of being torn between choices, which set off tantrums in the toddler year, she now expects to be able to draw in an adult—if she cries loud and long enough. When you hear her start, watch her eyes. Up until about age 2, her distress was internal. Her eyes showed it. She didn't "look for help." But a 2-year-old uses her eyes to "check out" her effect on those around her. A wise parent may prefer not to rush in to respond. Instead, urge her to fall back on her own resources to help herself. Encourage her to use her lovey or other toy for comfort in between storms, so that she'll be ready when she really needs it. When she can handle her own upset and resolve it herself, she will have learned a great deal about self-control.

Parents ask whether they can avoid tantrums by making light of each issue before the child gets too overwhelmed. Humor and being selective about picking battles are important. But she's bound to know when you are protecting her, and to feel undermined at times when she needs your encouragement to work it out herself. Tiptoeing on eggshells around a toddler surely won't help her learn to manage the tortured decision-making that leads to these tantrums. This step toward independence is a child's most important job in the second and third years.

Whining

From 2 to 5 years of age, a child who is bored or unable to amuse herself may turn to whining. She finds out quickly that whining is distasteful to her parents. If she is feeling sad, angry, or bored, it is a way to relieve those feelings. Her parent joins in battle, and she is no longer bored. "Mommy, mommy, I need you." The parent may feel rage welling up inside her and she can only respond with, "Stop it! I can't stand it!" I can remember how my younger brother and I would plot to make my mother blow up in frustration. It quickly became a goal all its own. Whining, though, can also become a means to an end, if a parent responds.

Discouraging Whining

1. Try to relieve her boredom with a "play date" or fun plans. But refer her also to her own ways of entertaining herself. She may need your help learning ways of entertaining herself. (Television will not teach her this.)
2. Label the child's whining to make her aware of her behavior: "You're whining."
3. Do not respond to what she says when she whines. Let her know that you are interested in what she has to say, but not while she's whining: "When you stop your whining, then we can talk. But not until you do."
4. When whining continues, walk away. But let her know that you are not abandoning her: "When you stop whining, I can come back."
5. When she stops, pick her up to hug her. But don't reward the whining.
6. Deal with your own anger and frustration somewhere else. It may be too rewarding to her to see you break down.
7. Always be sure she's not whining because she's ill or in pain.

BOOKS AND RESOURCES

Bibliography

Barr, R. G., Hopkins, B., and Green, J. A. "Crying as a Sign, a Symptom, and a Signal: Clinical, Emotional, and Developmental Aspects of Infant and Toddler Crying," in *Clinics in Developmental Medicine,* No. 152. London: Mac Keith Press, 2000.

Barr, R. G., St. James-Robert, I., and Keefe, M. R. *New Evidence on Unexplained Early Infant Crying: Its Origins, Nature, and Management.* Skillman, N.J.: Johnson and Johnson Pediatric Institute, 2001.

Barr, R. G., St. James-Robert, I., and Keefe, M. R. *Early Infant Crying: A Parent's Guide.* Skillman, N.J.: Johnson and Johnson Pediatric Institute, 2001.

Brazelton, T. B. "Crying in Infancy," in *Pediatrics* 29, 579–588 (1962).

Lester, B. M., and Boukydis, C. F. Z. *Infant Crying: Theoretical and Research Perspectives.* New York: Plenum Press, 1985.

Lester, B. M., Boukydis, C. F. Z., Garcia-Coll, C. T., Hole, W., and Peucker, M. "Infantile Colic: Acoustic Cry Characteristics,

Maternal Perception of Cry, and Temperament," in *Infant Behavior and Development* 15, 15–26 (1992).

Zeskind, P. S., and Barr, R. G. "Acoustic Characteristics of Naturally Occurring Cries of Infants with 'Colic'," in *Child Development* 68(3), 394–403 (June 1997).

Books for Parents

Brazelton, T. B. *Touchpoints: Your Child's Emotional and Behavioral Development.* Cambridge: Perseus Publishing, 1991.

Brazelton, T. B., and Sparrow, J. D. *Touchpoints Three to Six: Your Child's Emotional and Behavioral Development.* Cambridge: Perseus Publishing, 2001.

Stern, D. N. *Diary of a Baby.* New York: Basic Books, 1989.

Stern, D. N., and Bruschweiler-Stern, N. *The Birth of a Mother: How the Motherhood Experience Changes You Forever.* New York: Basic Books, 1998.

Woolf, A., Shane, H. C., and Kenna, M. A., Eds. *The Children's Hospital Guide to Your Child's Health and Development.* Cambridge: Perseus Publishing, 2000.

Resources for Parents

American Academy of Pediatrics
P.O. Box 927
Elk Grove Village, IL 60009
(847) 434-4000
www.aap.org

American Academy of Child and Adolescent Psychiatry
3615 Wisconsin Ave NW
Washington, D.C. 20016
(202) 966-7300
www.aacap.org

SIDS Resources

American SIDS Institute
2480 Windy Hill Road
Marietta, GA 30067
(800) 232-SIDS
www.sids.org

National SIDS Resource Center
2070 Chain Bridge Road, #450
Vienna, VA 22182
(800) 505-CRIB
www.sidscenter.org

Sudden Infant Death Syndrome Network
P.O. Box 520
Ledyard, CT 06339
(800) 339-7042 ext. 551
www.sids-network.org

On Postpartum Depression

Depression After Delivery, Inc.
91 East Somerset Street
Raritan, NJ 08869
(800) 944-4773
www.depressionafterdelivery.com

National Institutes of Mental Health
6001 Executive Blvd., Rm. 8184, MSC 9663
Bethesda, MD 20892-9663
(301) 443-4513
www.nimh.nih.gov

American Psychiatric Association
1400 K Street NW
Washington, D.C. 20005
(888) 357-7924
www.psych.org

On Infant Massage

Touch Research Institutes
University of Miami School of Medicine
P.O. Box 016820
Miami, FL 33101
(305) 243-6781
www.miami.edu/touch-research

Videotape on Calming Fussy Babies

Tim Healey, M.S., "Hush Little Baby: The Scientific, Systematic and Sensitive Way to Stop Excessive Crying." Kangaroo Kids, 1556 E. Katilla Ave., Anaheim, CA 92805; (714) 836-9036

On Feeling Pushed to the Edge

Parents Anonymous
675 W. Foothill Blvd., Suite 220
Claremont, CA 91711
(909) 621-6184
www.parentsanonymous.org

Acknowledgments

We would like to thank Richard and Tivia Kramer and the residents of the Harlem Children's Zone for having first urged us to write this concise, accessible book on a topic of the utmost importance to parents around the country, for without their vision it might never have been written. Thanks also go to Geoffrey Canada, Marilyn Joseph, Bart and Karen Lawson, David Saltzman, and Caressa Singleton, for their unwavering support for our work, and from whom we have learned so much. As always, we would again like to thank our editor, Merloyd Lawrence, for her wisdom and guidance. Finally, we wish to express our gratitude to our families, not only for their encouragement and patience, but also for the lessons they have taught us that we have sought to impart in this book.

Index

About the Authors

T. Berry Brazelton, M.D., founder of the Child Development Unit at Children's Hospital Boston, is Clinical Professor of Pediatrics Emeritus at Harvard Medical School. His many important and popular books include the internationally best-selling *Touchpoints* and *Infants and Mothers.* A practicing pediatrician for over forty-five years, Dr. Brazelton founded and co-directs two programs at Children's Hospital: the Brazelton Institute (www.brazelton–institute.com) and the Brazelton Touchpoints Center (www.touchpoints.org), which further his work nationally and around the world. Dr. Brazelton has also created the Brazelton Foundation (www.brazeltonfoundation.org) to support child development training for healthcare and educational professionals around the world.

Joshua D. Sparrow, M.D., Assistant Professor of Psychiatry at Harvard Medical School, is Supervisor of Inpatient Psychiatry at Children's Hospital Boston and Associate Director for Training at the Brazelton Touchpoints Center. He is the co-author, with Dr. Brazelton, of *Touchpoints Three to Six, Calming Your Fussy Baby: The Brazelton Way,* and *Discipline: The Brazelton Way.*